ULTIMATE LONGEVITY SUPPLEMENTS

How to Extend your Life Through Life Saving Supplements

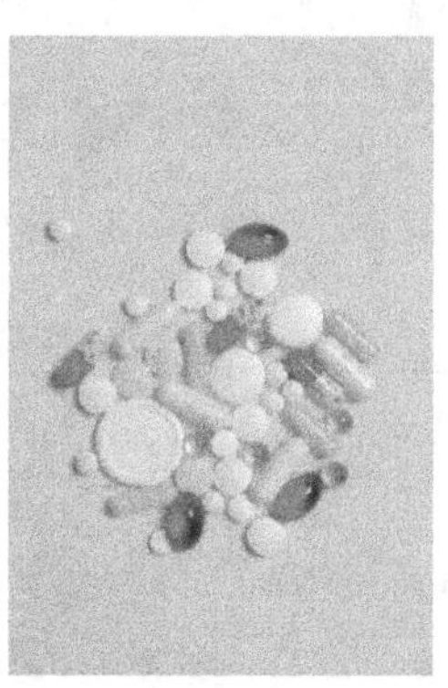

RICHARD R. LEON

OTHER BOOKS BY THE AUTHOR

SUPER EASY AIR FRYER COOKBOOK FOR SENIORS

REVERSING HEART DISEASE COOKBOOK

THE SECRET ART AND SCIENCE OF LONGEVITY

GLUCOSE INNOVATION

DIABETES DIET COOKBOOK FOR WOMEN 2023

DIABETES DIET COOKBOOK FOR MEN 2023

SMART DIABETIC DIET AFTER 50

WHAT IS OBESITY?

MEDITERRANEAN DIET COOKBOOK FOR TWO

KIDNEY DISEASE DIET COOKBOOK FOR BEGINNERS

TABLE OF CONTENT

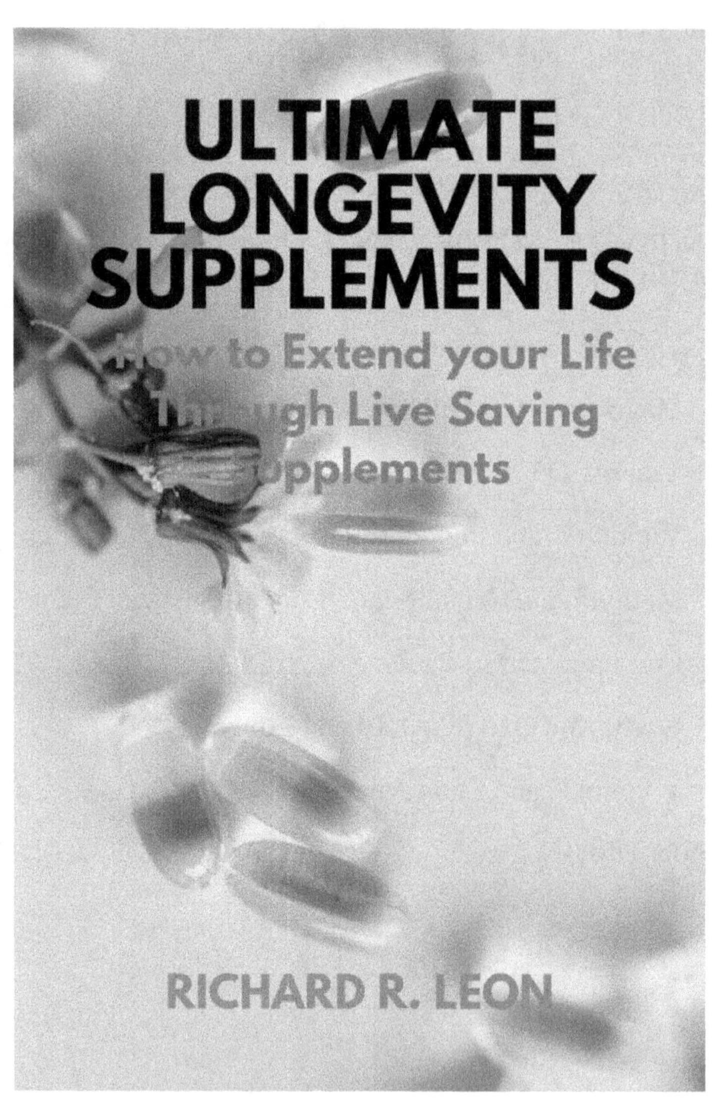

ULTIMATE
LONGEVITY
SUPPLEMENTS
How to Extend your Life
Through Live Saving
Supplements
RICHARD R. LEON

INTRODUCTION

Unlocking the Secret of Longevity

As scientific advances and improved healthcare extend our lifespans, the quest for longevity continues to capture our collective imagination. The desire to live a long and healthy life is an innate human ambition that transcends time, culture, and borders. It's an endeavor that has spawned countless explorations, experiments, and innovations, from the legendary quest for the fountain of youth to the latest advances in biotechnology and anti-aging research.

As we enter the 21st century, we face a unique moment in history. Science and technology are providing unprecedented insight into the biology of aging, providing insights into the mechanisms that determine lifespan and potential means of influencing lifespan. The science of longevity is no longer confined to myth or folklore but is now firmly established based on thorough research and empirical evidence.

This book is a journey into the fascinating field of longevity and an exploration of the science behind it. We will reveal the secrets of those who have overcome them and live incredible times, and give you the knowledge and tools you need to begin your journey to a longer, healthier life.

In the following pages, we will delve into the potential of supplements for longevity. We explore their impact on the aging process with the latest research on antioxidants, telomere support, NAD precursors, anti-inflammatory compounds, and mitochondrial health.

From increasing vitality and cognitive function to reducing chronic disease, you'll discover the potential benefits of adopting a longevity-focused lifestyle.

this book isn't just about the latest scientific breakthroughs or a list of supplements that promise longevity. It also highlights the importance of But a holistic approach to health and well-being. We discuss the importance of physical activity, how stress affects aging, the importance of good sleep, and the social connections that improve your life.

Longevity is not a one-dimensional concept. It is a personal journey. The choices you make, the knowledge you acquire, and the lifestyle you adopt shape your unique path to a long and healthy life. We hope this book will guide you, pave the way for your future, give you the information you need to make informed decisions and inspire you to take control of your longevity journey.

The pursuit of longevity is not an individual endeavor. It is a shared journey that connects us in time and space. Join us on this extraordinary expedition to discover the secret to longevity, embrace the wonderful opportunities that await us, and live life to the fullest.

LONGEVITY SUPPLEMENTS THAT CAN EXTEND YOUR LIFE

Fish Oil Capsules and Longevity

Nourish Your Way to a Healthier, Longer Life: In recent years, fish oil capsules have received a lot of attention not only for their potential to support overall health but also for their association with longevity. Rich in omega-3 essential fatty acids, this supplement has been the subject of extensive research and has proven to be a promising ally in the pursuit of a long and healthy life.

Omega-3 fatty acids are a group of polyunsaturated fats that the human body needs and must obtain through diet or supplements. Fish oil is a known source of two essential omega-3 fatty acids: eicosapentaenoic acid (EPA) and docosahexaenoic acid (DHA). These fatty acids play an important role in a variety of bodily processes and have been linked to several health benefits related to longevity.

Cardiovascular health: One of the most well-known benefits of fish oil is its positive effect on heart health. Omega-3 fatty acids help lower triglyceride levels, lower blood pressure, and reduce the risk of heart disease. Maintaining a healthy heart is fundamental to longevity as it promotes a long and active life.

Brain health: The cognitive benefits of omega-3 fatty acids are also notable.

In particular, DHA is an important part of brain cell membranes. Studies have shown that regular consumption of fish oil can improve quality of life as you age, supporting cognitive function and reducing the risk of cognitive decline later in life. Inflammation and

Chronic Disease: Chronic inflammation is a common feature of many age-related diseases. Omega-3 fatty acids are known for their anti-inflammatory properties and may reduce the risk of developing chronic diseases such as arthritis, diabetes, and some cancers.

Cellular aging: Fish oil can also have a positive effect on cellular aging. As humans age, the protective caps known as telomeres on the ends of chromosomes shorten. Reduced telomere length is linked to cellular aging and a higher chance of developing age-related illnesses. Some studies suggest that omega-3 fatty acids may help maintain telomere length, slowing the aging process at the cellular level.

Fish oil capsules offer many potential benefits for longevity, but it is important to remember that the quality and purity of the supplement are important. Not all fish oil supplements are created equal, and it's best to choose a high-quality version free of contaminants such as heavy metals and toxins.

It is also important to remember that supplements should complement a balanced diet and a healthy lifestyle. Longevity is a multi-faceted journey that includes elements such as a nutritious diet, regular exercise, stress management, and social relationships.

Fish oil capsules can be a valuable addition to this journey, but they work best when combined with a holistic approach to health and wellness.

In conclusion, fish oil capsules rich in omega-3 fatty acids are a valuable tool in the quest for longevity. The potential benefits for heart health, brain function, reduced inflammation, and cellular aging make it an attractive option for people who want to live a longer, healthier life. When chosen wisely and used as part of an overall health strategy, fish oil supplements can play a truly important role in your journey to a more vibrant and longer life.

Magnesium Capsules and Longevity

Hidden Gems for a Healthy and Long Life: In the ever-evolving landscape of supplements designed to promote longevity and health, magnesium capsules have emerged as an unsung hero. This common mineral is essential for the proper functioning of the human body and has been linked to several health benefits, making it a potential ally in the pursuit of a long and healthy life.

Magnesium is involved in over 300 biochemical reactions in the body and contributes to the health and maintenance of a variety of systems and functions.

Magnesium capsules can play an important role in longevity.One.

Cardiovascular Health: Magnesium is known for its ability to support cardiovascular health. It helps regulate blood pressure, maintain a healthy heartbeat, and improve the elasticity of blood vessels.

These measures reduce the risk of high blood pressure and reduce the likelihood of developing heart disease, a key contributor to longevity.

Bone health: Adequate magnesium strengthens bones. It helps with calcium absorption and metabolism, increases bone density, and reduces the risk of fractures and osteoporosis, which can be life-limiting later in life. Muscle and nerve function: Magnesium is necessary for the proper functioning of muscles and nerves. It plays an important role in muscle contraction and relaxation, as well as in nerve signal transmission. Maintaining healthy muscle and nerve function is essential for overall mobility and quality of life as you age.

Sleep quality: Good sleep is essential for longevity, and magnesium can help improve sleep quality. It helps relax muscles and increase quality, making it easier to fall asleep and stay asleep. Quality sleep is associated with many health benefits, including improved cognitive function and support of the immune system.

Antioxidant protection: Magnesium participates in the body's antioxidant defense system and helps reduce oxidative stress and inflammation. Reducing oxidative stress is essential for slowing the aging process and reducing the risk of age-related diseases.

Blood sugar control: Keeping blood sugar levels stable is important for longevity. Magnesium helps regulate insulin and blood sugar levels, reducing the risk of type 2 diabetes and related complications.

Stress Management: Chronic stress is known to accelerate aging. Magnesium helps the body manage stress by supporting the adrenal glands and promoting relaxation.

Magnesium capsules offer potential longevity benefits, but it's important to note that not all supplements are created equal. Magnesium supplements can vary in quality and bioavailability, so it's important to choose a high-quality product that fits your needs.

In particular, magnesium is best used as part of a holistic approach to health and longevity. A balanced lifestyle that includes magnesium-rich foods such as green leafy vegetables, nuts, seeds, and whole grains in your diet, along with regular exercise and stress management, will maximize the benefits of magnesium supplementation.

Simply put, magnesium capsules are a hidden gem in the world of longevity supplements. Its potential to support cardiovascular health, bone strength, muscle and nerve function, sleep quality, antioxidant protection, glycemic control, and stress management make it a valuable addition to the pursuit of a long and healthy life. When combined with a holistic approach to wellness, magnesium capsules shine as the basic foundation for a vibrant and extended life.

Vitamin D Capsules and Longevity

Light the Path to a Healthier and Longer Life: In the pursuit of a long and healthy life, no nutrient receives more attention than vitamin D. Vitamin D capsules, often called the "sunshine vitamin," have become an essential part of the pursuit of longevity and wellness.

This versatile vitamin plays an important role in many body processes and is associated with numerous health benefits that may be the key to extending our lifespan.

Vitamin D is unique among vitamins in that it can be produced in the body when the skin is exposed to sunlight, or it can be obtained through diet or supplements. Important features include:.

Bone health: Vitamin D is known to play an important role in calcium absorption and bone metabolism. Adequate intake of this vitamin is essential for maintaining strong bones and reducing the risk of osteoporosis, fractures, and bone-related problems later in life, which greatly affect quality of life.

Immune System Support: Vitamin D strengthens both innate and adaptive immune responses. It reduces the risk of infectious diseases and strengthens the body's defense against various diseases, helping to maintain health and resistance to aging.

Cardiovascular health: Vitamin D also has a positive effect on heart health. Studies have shown that adequate levels of vitamin D are associated with a reduced risk of cardiovascular disease, including high blood pressure, atherosclerosis, and heart attacks.

Cognitive function: Emerging research suggests that vitamin D may play a role in supporting cognitive function and reducing the risk of cognitive decline. This is essential for improving your quality of life as you age.

Anti-inflammatory effects: Chronic inflammation is a common feature of many age-related diseases.

Vitamin D has anti-inflammatory properties that help reduce inflammation and reduce the risk of age-related diseases.

Mood and mental health: Adequate levels of vitamin D are associated with improved mood and mental health. Mental health is such an important part of overall well-being and longevity that vitamin D's effects in this area are unique.

However, vitamin D supplementation is especially important for people with limited exposure to sunlight, such as those who live in northern latitudes or have limited outdoor activities. Additionally, the body's ability to synthesize vitamin D from sunlight declines with age, making supplementation even more important for older adults.

As with all supplements, it is important to ensure the quality and purity of your vitamin D capsules. You should consult your doctor for advice on proper dosage.

Vitamin D capsules are a promising ally in the quest for longevity and support bone health, immune system function, cardiovascular health, cognitive vitality, and emotional balance. By incorporating these capsules into a comprehensive health and longevity strategy, we can pave the way to a brighter, longer life.

Vitamin E and longevity

Antioxidant protection for a healthy and long life: In the quest for a longer, healthier life, vitamin E plays a key role in the ever-expanding world of nutritional science. Known for its role in protecting cells from oxidative damage, this fat-soluble antioxidant has become popular for its potential effects on longevity.

Vitamin E is composed of several compounds, with alpha-tocopherol being the most biologically active form. How vitamin E relates to longevity and overall well-being:

Antioxidant Protection: Oxidative stress, caused by an imbalance of harmful free radicals and antioxidants in the body, is a major cause of aging and age-related diseases. As a potent antioxidant, vitamin E scavenges free radicals and shields cells from harm. Being protected like this helps people live long, healthy lives.

Heart health: One of the main causes of death globally is cardiovascular disease. Vitamin E is thought to support heart health by preventing the oxidation of low-density lipoprotein (LDL) cholesterol, a major risk factor for heart disease. By reducing the risk of atherosclerosis and blood clots, vitamin E helps maintain a healthy heart and prolong life.

Cognitive function: Cognitive decline and neurodegenerative diseases can have a significant impact on quality of life later in life. The antioxidant properties of vitamin E may support cognitive function, reducing the risk of diseases such as Alzheimer's disease and dementia.

Supports the immune system: A strong immune system is essential to fight infections and stay healthy as you age. Vitamin E helps boost immune function, which is important for a long and active life.

Skin health: Visible signs of aging, such as wrinkles and age spots, are often caused by damage to the skin caused by oxidative stress. Vitamin E protects your skin from this damage, helping you maintain a youthful appearance and boost your confidence as you age.

Eye Health: Poor vision is a common problem among the aging population. Vitamin E helps reduce the risk of age-related eye diseases such as macular degeneration and cataracts by protecting the eye's delicate tissues from oxidative damage.

Cellular longevity: Vitamin E's ability to reduce oxidative stress reaches the cellular level, slowing the aging process and reducing the risk of age-related diseases.

As with all supplements, the quality and form of vitamin E are important. Vitamin E comes in many forms, but alpha-tocopherol is the most biologically active. Excessive amounts of vitamin E are not suitable for everyone and can cause side effects, so it is advisable to consult a doctor.

Incorporating vitamin E into a holistic approach to health and longevity, including a balanced diet, regular exercise, stress management, and social activity, can significantly improve your well-being and extend your life. Vitamin E acts as a protective shield that protects the body from the ravages of time and promotes a long, healthy, and fulfilling life.

Methylfolate Capsules and Longevity

Accelerate Your Journey to a Healthier and Longer Life: In the quest for longevity and an active, healthy life, methylfolate capsules are gaining popularity as a supplement that can make a big difference. Methylfolate, also known as L-methylfolate or 5-MTHF, is the naturally active form of folic acid. Its importance in promoting longevity is based on its central role in several important body functions. Methylfolate is essential for several processes, including DNA synthesis and repair, neurotransmitter regulation, and homocysteine metabolism.

Here's how methylfolate capsules can contribute to a longer, healthier life

Cardiovascular Health: Maintaining healthy homocysteine levels is essential for heart health. Elevated homocysteine is a known risk factor for cardiovascular disease, including atherosclerosis and stroke. Methylfolate helps promote a healthy heart by metabolizing and lowering homocysteine levels.

Cognitive function: Adequate levels of methylfolate are associated with improved cognitive function, especially in older adults. It plays an important role in regulating neurotransmitters that are important for maintaining memory, focus, and mental agility as we age.

DNA Integrity: Methylfolate is essential for DNA synthesis and repair. Maintaining the integrity of genetic material is essential for reducing the risk of age-related diseases, including some cancers.

Mood and emotional well-being: Methylfolate is involved in the synthesis of mood-regulating neurotransmitters such as serotonin and dopamine. Adequate levels of methylfolate help maintain emotional balance and mental health and improve the overall quality of life in old age.

Health genivillery: For those who intend to make live children later, methylfolli acid is important for the prevention of neurological defects during pregnancy, which is increasingly relevant as an individual extends the fertile year.

Energy and Vitality: Methylfolate promotes energy production at the cellular level. Maintaining optimal energy levels is essential to getting active, staying active, and living a longer, more fulfilling life.

It is important to remember that many people have genetic changes that affect their ability to convert folic acid to its active form, methylfolate. Methylfolate supplementation is especially important for these people. In addition, it is necessary to ensure the quality and cleanliness of methyl folic acid capsules.

It is recommended to recommend medical service providers for effective doses and personal interaction guidelines for other drugs.

Methylfolate capsules serve as a valuable resource in the quest for longevity, supporting cardiovascular health, cognitive function, DNA integrity, emotional well-being, and reproductive health. By combining these capsules in a holistic approach to health and longevity, people can pave the way for a brighter and longer life.

Curcumin and Longevity

Using the Golden Spice of Life: In the ever-evolving environment of longevity and health, curcumin, the bioactive compound in turmeric, is receiving a lot of attention. Revered for its bright golden color and health benefits, curcumin is emerging as a powerful tool for a long and healthy life.

Curcumin, a polyphenol with powerful antioxidant and anti-inflammatory properties, has been a staple in traditional medicine for centuries. Curcumin has been linked to longevity.

Anti-inflammatory and antioxidant power: Chronic inflammation and oxidative stress are key factors in the aging process and the development of age-related diseases. Curcumin, with its powerful anti-inflammatory and antioxidant properties, helps block this process and reduce the risk of age-related diseases.

Brain health: Cognitive decline is a major concern with aging, and curcumin shows promise in this area. It is associated with improved cognitive function and a reduced risk of neurodegenerative diseases such as Alzheimer's disease. Maintaining mental clarity and brain health is essential to living a prolonged, high-quality life..

Cardiovascular Support: Heart health is the foundation of a long life. Curcumin is known to improve cardiovascular health by reducing risk factors associated with heart disease, such as high blood pressure, high cholesterol, and atherosclerosis.

Joint Health: Mobility and an active lifestyle are essential for a full and extended life. Curcumin can help relieve joint pain and stiffness, improve conditions such as arthritis, and promote an active lifestyle later in life.

Cellular Longevity: Curcumin has been shown to affect cellular processes associated with longevity, including activation of genes associated with longevity and extended cellular lifespan. This presents an exciting opportunity to slow the aging process at the cellular level.

Cancer prevention: Chronic inflammation and oxidative stress contribute to the development of cancer. Curcumin's anti-inflammatory and antioxidant properties help reduce the risk of cancer and prevent life-threatening diseases.

Gut Health: A healthy gut is the foundation of your overall well-being. Curcumin improves gut health by maintaining the balance of beneficial gut bacteria and reducing inflammation, which plays an important role in improving quality of life and longevity.

As with all supplements, the quality and purity of curcumin capsules are very important. The bioavailability of curcumin can be limited, so choosing a formula that enhances absorption is recommended.

Adding curcumin to a holistic approach to health and longevity, along with a balanced diet, regular exercise, stress management, and social activity can provide significant benefits. Often referred to as the "herb of life", curcumin offers comprehensive tools in the pursuit of a long, healthy, and vibrant life.

Coenzyme Q10 (CoQ10) and Longevity

Promote Your Journey to a Healthier, Longer Life: In your pursuit of a long and healthy life, focus on Coenzyme Q10, also known as CoQ10. This natural compound, found in every cell of the human body, becomes a key element in the quest for longevity, unlocking the potential to improve well-being and prolong old age.

CoQ10 serves as an important component in the production of adenosine triphosphate (ATP), the energy currency of our cells. This important role, along with its powerful antioxidant properties, makes CoQ10 an important molecule in the context of longevity. CoQ10 shows a correlation between health and longevity.

Energy production: As we age, cellular energy production declines, which can lead to fatigue and decreased vitality. CoQ10 plays a central role in the mitochondrial respiratory chain and ensures efficient ATP synthesis. By optimizing energy production, CoQ10 helps maintain physical and mental strength and improves overall quality of life.

Cardiovascular health: Heart health is the foundation of a long life. CoQ10 is an essential nutrient for the heart muscle and helps maintain the integrity of heart tissue and improve blood circulation. Its antioxidant properties help reduce oxidative stress in the cardiovascular system, reduce the risk of heart disease, and prolong life.

Antioxidant protection: Oxidative stress, characterized by an imbalance of free radicals and antioxidants in the body, is a major factor in aging and age-related diseases. CoQ10's powerful antioxidant properties prevent oxidative damage, protect cells from damage, and reduce the risk of several diseases.

Cognitive function: Cognitive decline and neurodegenerative diseases can have a significant impact on quality of life as you age. CoQ10 may support cognitive function by promoting healthy circulation, reducing oxidative stress, and improving overall brain cell viability.

Supports the Immune System: A strong immune system is essential to stay healthy and prolong life. CoQ10 has been linked to improved immune function, which is essential for fighting infection and supporting overall well-being.

Cellular Longevity: The antioxidant effects of CoQ10 reach the cellular level, helping to protect cells from oxidative damage and reduce the risk of age-related diseases. This contributes to a long and healthy life.

As with all supplements, the quality and bioavailability of CoQ10 is of utmost importance. A variety of formulations and dosages are available, and consultation with a healthcare professional can help determine the most appropriate option based on your individual needs and health concerns.

Adding CoQ10 to a holistic approach to health and longevity that includes a balanced diet, regular exercise, stress management, and social activity can significantly improve your well-being and extend your golden years. CoQ10 acts as a source of cellular energy, providing more vitality and longer life.

Vitamin C and Longevity

The Timeless Elixir of Health and Vitality: A nutrient that has stood the test of time as a powerful ally in the pursuit of a long and healthy life is vitamin C. Also known as ascorbic acid, this water-soluble vitamin is known to have profound effects and consequences on human health.

The possibility of extending the golden age. As a cornerstone of nutritional science, the importance of vitamin C in promoting longevity cannot be overstated.

Here's how vitamin C is linked to a healthy and long life. One.

Antioxidant power: Oxidative stress, characterized by an imbalance of harmful free radicals and antioxidants in the body, is a major cause of aging and age-related diseases. Vitamin C is a powerful antioxidant that fights free radicals, protects cells from damage, and reduces the risk of various health problems.

Supports the Immune System: A strong immune system is essential to fight infections and stay healthy as you age. Vitamin C plays an important role in the functioning of the immune system and can play an important role in extending life by increasing the body's ability to fight infection and disease.

Heart health: Cardiovascular disease is one of the leading causes of death worldwide. The antioxidant properties of vitamin C help reduce oxidative stress in the cardiovascular system, reducing the risk of heart disease, high blood pressure, and atherosclerosis, leading to a healthier heart and longer life expectancy.

Skin health: Visible signs of aging, such as wrinkles and age spots, are often caused by skin damage caused by oxidative stress. Vitamin C is essential for collagen synthesis. Collagen synthesis is essential for maintaining skin elasticity, preventing premature aging, maintaining a youthful appearance, and increasing confidence in later life.

Cognitive function: Cognitive decline and neurodegenerative diseases can have a significant impact on the quality of life as you age. Vitamin C supports cognitive function, reduces the risk of diseases such as Alzheimer's disease, promotes mental clarity, and extends life.

Eye Health: Poor vision is a common problem among the aging population. Vitamin C can reduce the risk of age-related eye diseases such as macular degeneration and cataracts by protecting the eye's sensitive tissue from oxidative damage.

Wound Healing: The ability to heal wounds and surgeries becomes more important as we age. Vitamin C is essential for the production of collagen, the main component of skin, connective tissue, and blood vessels. Maintaining adequate levels of vitamin C can support the body's healing and regenerative abilities and improve quality of life.

As with all supplements, the quality and purity of vitamin C are very important. There are many different forms, including ascorbic acid and buffered vitamin C, and consultation with a healthcare professional can help determine the most appropriate option based on your individual needs and health concerns.

Adding vitamin C to a holistic approach to health and longevity, along with a balanced diet, regular exercise, stress management, and social activity, can significantly improve your well-being and extend your golden years. Vitamin C acts as a timeless elixir of health and vitality, promoting the journey to a longer and healthier life.

CONCLUSION

Choosing supplements in the world of health and longevity can be overwhelming. From fish oil to methyl folate, vitamin D, coenzyme Q10, and more, each supplement has a unique promise to support a long, healthy life.

While the potential of these supplements is great, it is important to remember that they are only one piece of the longevity puzzle. Pursuing a more active and longer life is a multi-faceted journey. It is important not only to choose your supplements carefully but also to take a holistic approach to your health.

A balanced, nutrient-dense diet, regular physical activity, effective stress management, good sleep, and meaningful social relationships are all essential components of the equation.

Supplements like the ones we studied can benefit heart health, cognitive function, immune system stability, and more. Providing support can serve as a valuable tool in this journey.

However, it is important to use it wisely and ensure the quality and purity of the supplements you choose. We recommend that you consult with your doctor to determine which supplement is best for your individual needs and to consider potential interactions with medications or pre-existing health conditions.

In conclusion, the supplements we investigated, from vitamin C to CoQ10, offer exciting possibilities for improving health and extending life. When combined with a holistic approach to wellness, it becomes an essential component in the pursuit of a long, healthy, and fulfilling life. Ultimately, the journey to longevity is a personal journey, and by taking these supplements and adopting a holistic lifestyle, we embrace the promise of a long and bright future and empower ourselves to live life to the fullest.

9 798887 124 0632